For Ladies Only
Dedicated to the Color Pink

By Ayin M. Adams

Copyright © 2010 by Ayin M. Adams

ISBN-13
978-0-9841228-4-4

ISBN-10
0-9841228-4-2

First Edition: March 2011

Cover Idea by Ayin M. Adams

Cover Design by Junior's Digital Designs

Typesetting by Saforabu Graphix

Author's Photo by Terri Rainey

Photo credits inside book supplied by Kathryn Waddell Takara, Terri Rainey and Ayin Adams

Published by PACIFIC RAVEN PRESS

P.O. Box 678 Ka`a`awa, Hawai`i 96730

www.pacificravenpress.com

email: pacificravenpress@gmail.com

Telephone: 1-808-276-6864 USA

Fax number: 1-808-237-8974 USA

Published in the United States of America

Printed in USA

Books by Ayin M. Adams

African Americans In Hawai`i: A Search For Identity

The Woods Deep Inside Me

Walking In Sappho's Garden

Walking Through My Fire

Books edited by Ayin M. Adams

Climbing A Rainbow of Dreams

Butterflies Blossom

From Dawn To Dusk

Graffiti Dreams

Dedication

To all women, sisters, daughters, friends, families, mothers, grandmothers, and men who have experienced cancer.

Acknowledgements

I want to thank Spirit for allowing my heart to open up, my ears to hear the voices calling out to me, and my willingness to go forward in a tangible endearing way. I thank my beloved late parents Robert & Virginia Adams, Kathryn Waddell Takara, Frieda Groffy, Mary Denise Wagner, Mrs. Lee, Claire Gibo, Hattie Childs, Terri Rainey, my sisters Christine & Linda Adams, Lorraine Nole-Rippy, Pat Matsumoto, Sandra Shawhan, Sodengi C. Orimaladi Mills, sisters around the globe, the American Cancer Society, Junior Mclean, Stacy Comer, and the many strong men who have balanced their inner selves with their outer, while honoring the divine feminine. You are the strong and gifted ones.

Thank you all!

Preface

Throughout the entirety of this epic poem on Breast Cancer, I aim to take you on an emotional roller coaster and end with a hope for healing.

The book is a long ride that begins at birth, and takes a short halt at all the stations through childhood, girl, adolescence, young lady, young woman, young adult, woman, and finally, the ride takes you forward to and through mature womanhood!

Breasts become like an alter ego that you can talk to, that you can confide in, that you can love, and that you can adore. I have attempted to write this poem with a touch of humor and also with a touch of tenderness. Within the pages, there is also the real fear, the rough pain, denial, rebellion, the out-spoken courage, and the frailty of the struggle.

Most women have known or know within their circle of family and friends, a sister who is confronted with the reality of fighting the dragon! Some women exit their fight as winners, but all too often, many make their exit from life, thus, succumbing to the insidious killer disease.

The empathy towards the havoc that the disease causes to the lives of women, (and sometimes men) and their families comes through every stanza of the poem and feels like a healing patch over a deep scar!

For example, The line "The griefs of my own lie heavy in my breasts" moves in and out like a rhythmic dance of the African Djembe drums. The beat often calls us back to the heartbeat of life, the fight for survival, the will to win, the thrust to push forward towards healing in spite of the appearances of hopelessness and despair which surround us in everyday life. This is the first beat we hear in our mother's womb. This heartbeat is the first beat that restores us, sacredly sustains us, and encourages us to hope for more life.

"The griefs of my own lie heavy in my breasts," is a return to the call of the drum beat and life, the call of woman finally releasing her own inner imprisoned splendour!

Introduction

For Ladies Only: Dedicated to the Color Pink is a moving and revealing small book in poetic verse about a major health problem, breast cancer, from a unique personal perspective of the birth, development and growth of breasts. It is a healing sometimes humorous journey from dawn to night, from birth to death in the shadow of cancer, a group of diseases that is often still uncontrollable cellular growth affecting different parts of the body, but in women most often the breasts.

Ayin Adams personifies breasts as dear and intimate friends who are as essential as organs, as necessary as limbs, as nurturing as companions that accompany one through each of life's stages, rituals, processes. Her focus is on the affirmation of breasts, will, the unity of women in gender/health issues ending in a declaration of hope for a cure and an affirmation of the joys of life's intimate moments. An empowering, insightful book.

Kathryn Waddell Takara, PhD.
2010 American Book Award Winner of Pacific Raven: Hawai`i Poems

For Ladies Only
Dedicated to the Color Pink

By Ayin M. Adams

For Ladies Only

Dedicated to the Color Pink

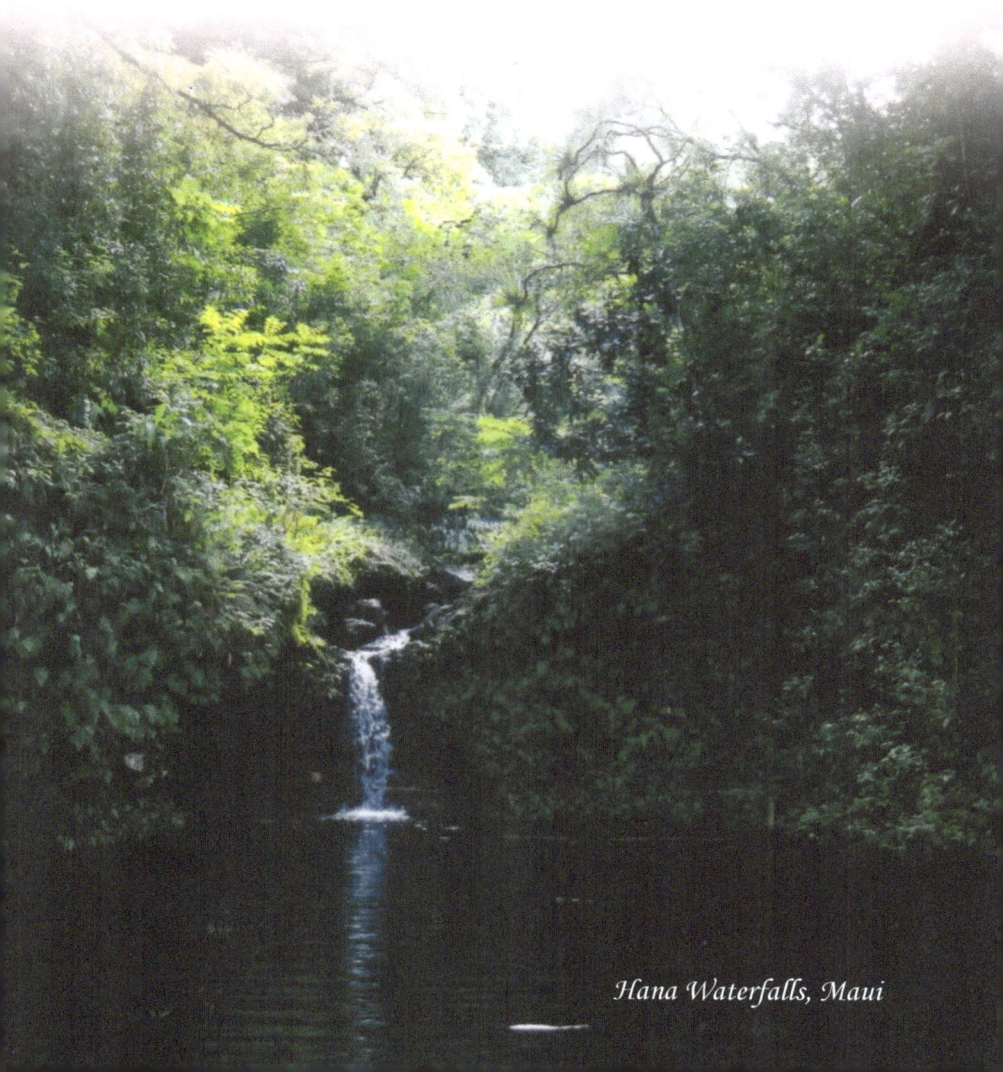

Mother said you were, "Little like door knobs
bright, round and brown."
An exciting time for me
that marked the growth of development
into a world later where anxiousness

would be replaced by worries.

Hana Waterfalls, Maui

Then came the time I avoided pink.
I didn't want pink any more.
I didn't want pink as a painful reminder.
I didn't want pink categorized
as a sorority for sisters.
I didn't want pink labeled for a specific gender.
I didn't want pink to remind me of
the words, "For Ladies Only."
I didn't want pink forever
stigmatized as a ribbon.
I didn't want pink as a sign of failing health.

Kanaha Beach State Park, Maui

Pink no longer held the cherished
childhood fantasies, neither make-believe memories
nor, the meaning of why little girls
loved pink barrettes, dolls and stockings.

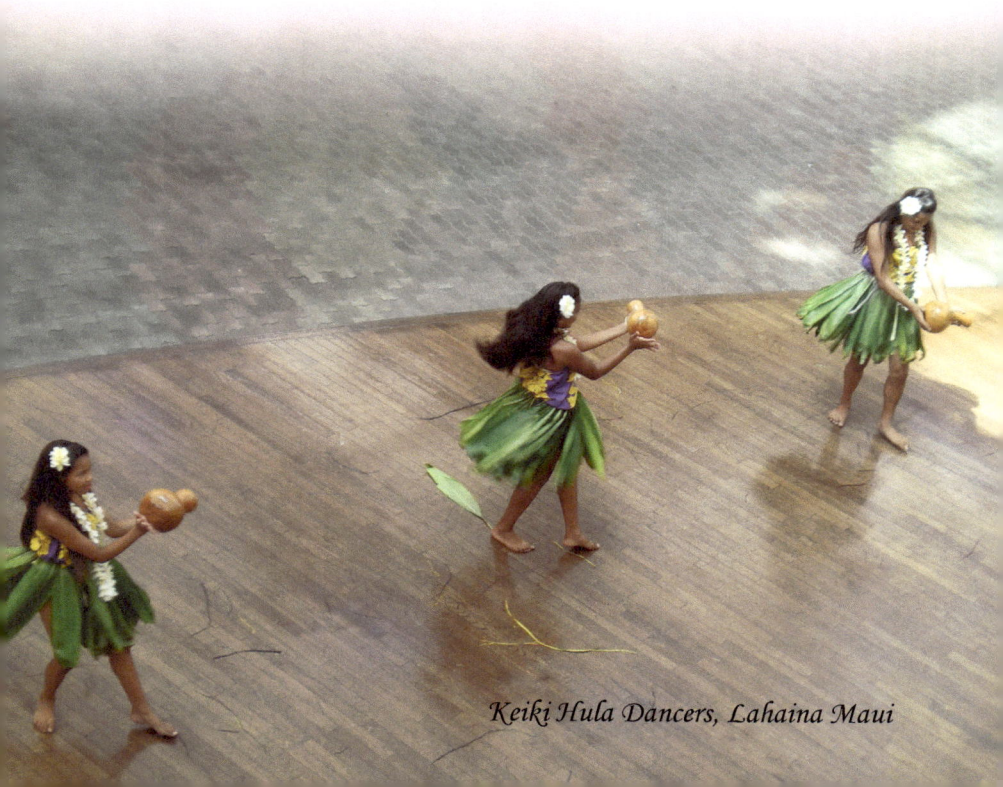

Keiki Hula Dancers, Lahaina Maui

Pretty little door knobs.
They would increase in size
with the passing of birthdays and
growth into maturity,
punctuated by cramps, bloatedness,
and menstrual cycles.

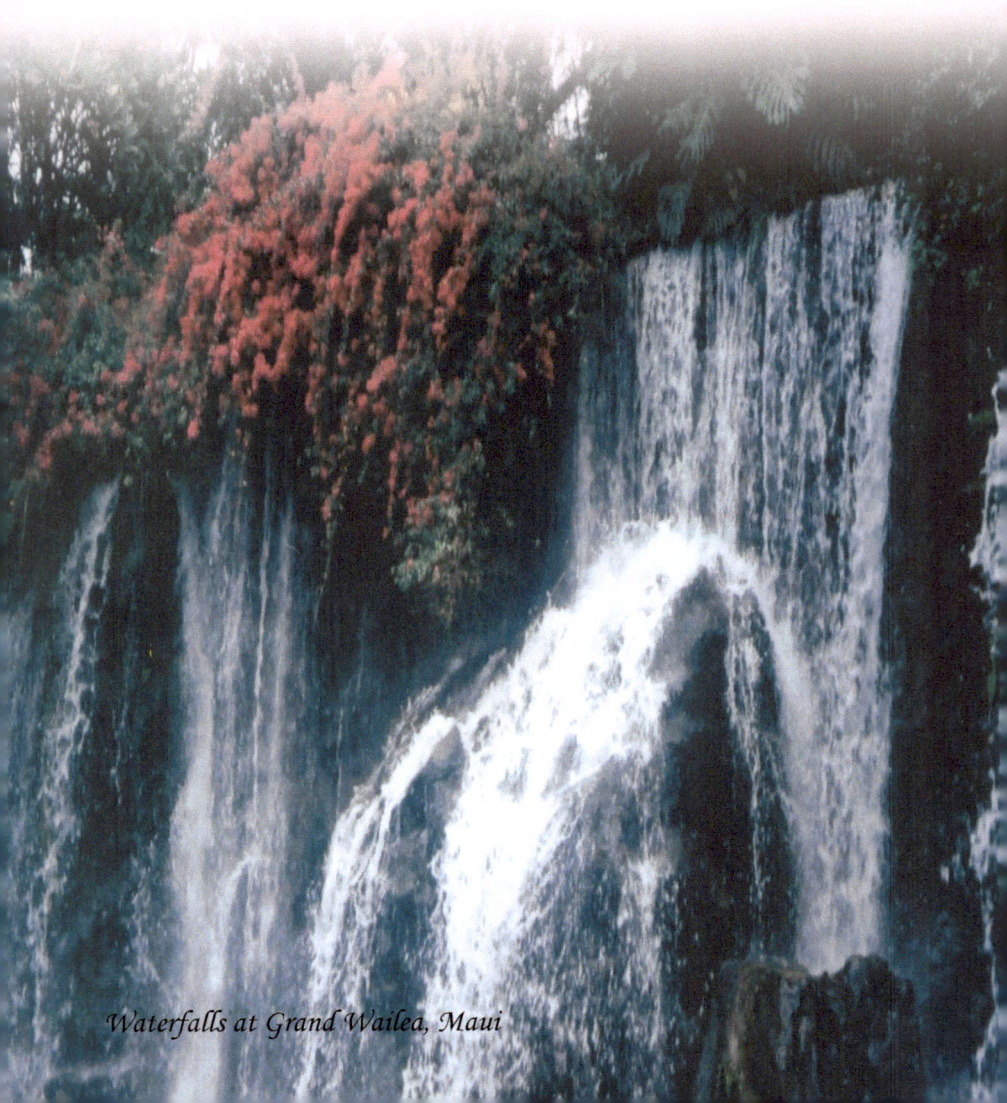

Waterfalls at Grand Wailea, Maui

Pretty precious doorknobs
I took them to bed every night
faithful, faithful as a doting lover
I held them when my body ached sorely
sang lullabies to wash away the sadness
rubbed my belly when dreams appeared frightening

comforted them in my loneliness when they were not touched.

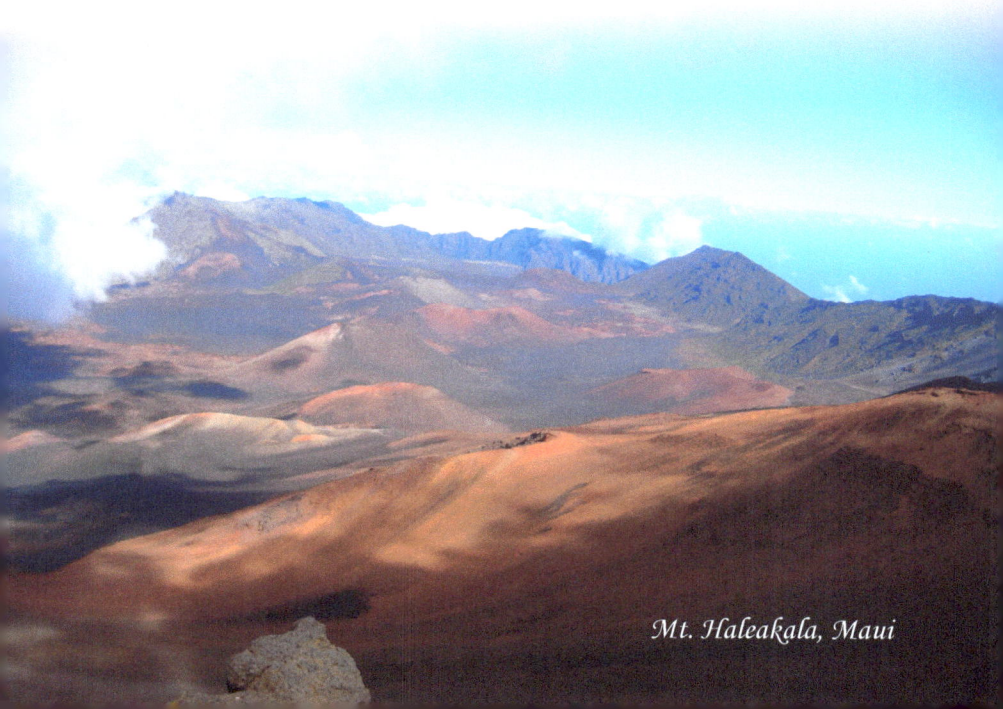

Mt. Haleakala, Maui

I laughed at them, delighted in their posturing
--erect--
standing at the position of attention
saluting the vibrancy of youth
ever growing more plump and supple.

Coconut Tree

Then, mysteriously, painstakingly,
they began to withdraw, disappearing
slowly…inverting. My refusal to leave
their betrayal to give me milk,
silky substance that I needed
to claim and affirm my womanhood.
Silky substance that I needed to need me!
Silky substance that made me feel proud,
look beautiful and helped me to fake it
even when I was not at my best!
I needed them!   I needed me!

Heulo Lookout, Maui

Suddenly I was
sneaking, blundering, groping,
hiding, wandering in the vast darkness of despair.
I no longer wanted to dance naked
in front of the waiting mesmerizing mirror.

Sunset on Kauai

Exiting the black shower, I began to hide in shadows.
Half-hazard attempts to dry myself failed,
leaving a trail of broken tears on the damp floor
slippery as eels, that I could never mop up
nor refrain from running astray.

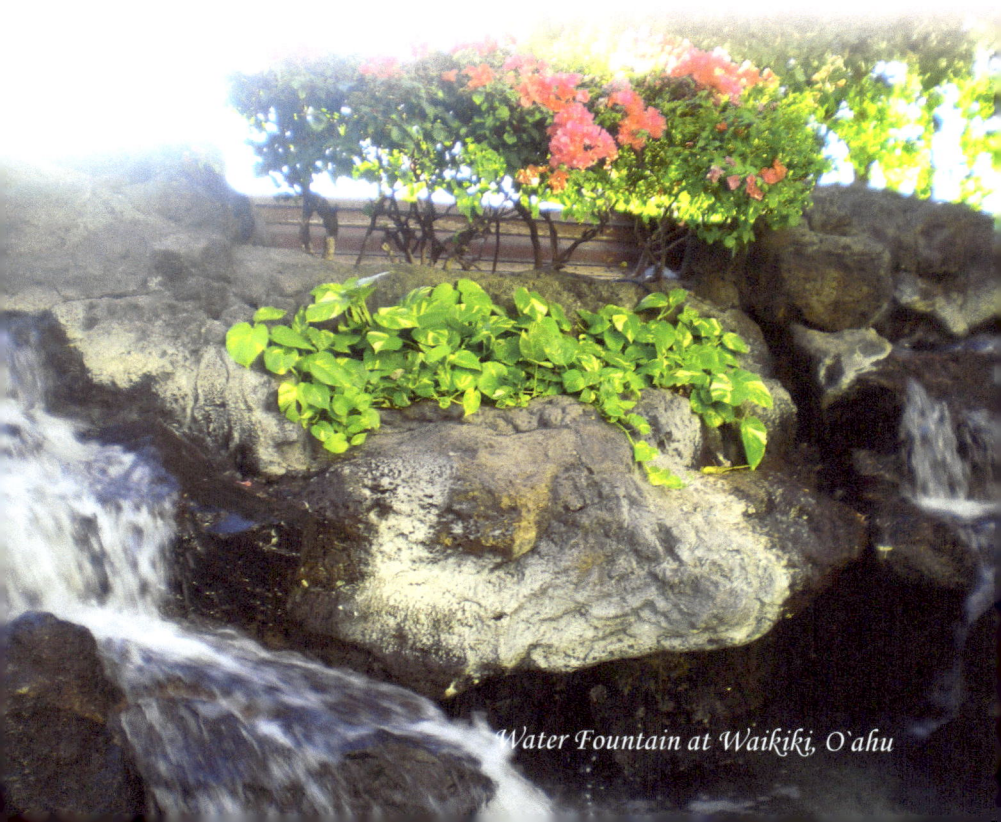

Water Fountain at Waikiki, O`ahu

My breasts distanced themselves from me,
becoming unfamiliar, more shady,
somber, cold, rigid,
as if we could server our lives completely
totally, without feeling abandoned!
I hungered, isolated,
numbness came to claim me.

Mt. Haleakala Crater, Maui

Descending,
        Descending,
                Descending,
into the bleak world
of desolate lives to try to live
where misty veils cling
to the most unnatural parts of ourselves
hauntingly!

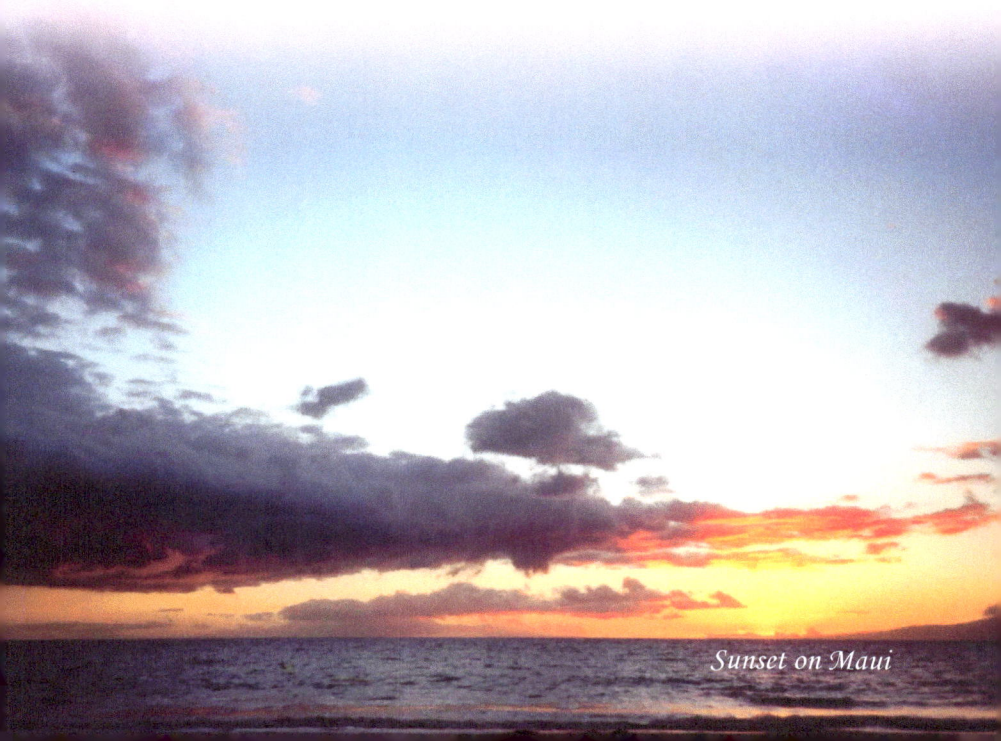

Sunset on Maui

The griefs of my own lie heavy in my breasts.
Again and again and again
over and over and over again
slowly one (of them) grew larger
sickness embedded
like journalists in war
hard as an orange, clean as a bald head
while the other twin remained untouched
unscathed by the hostile legions of contamination
that grew next to the heart we once called home.
The griefs of my own lie heavy in my breasts!

Ancient Streams At Sacred Iao Valley, Maui

How could I go on and live?
Life—without them--
could crawl to a slow drag—then stop
like water in Winter.
Ice.
Frozen.
The griefs of my own lie heavy in my breasts!

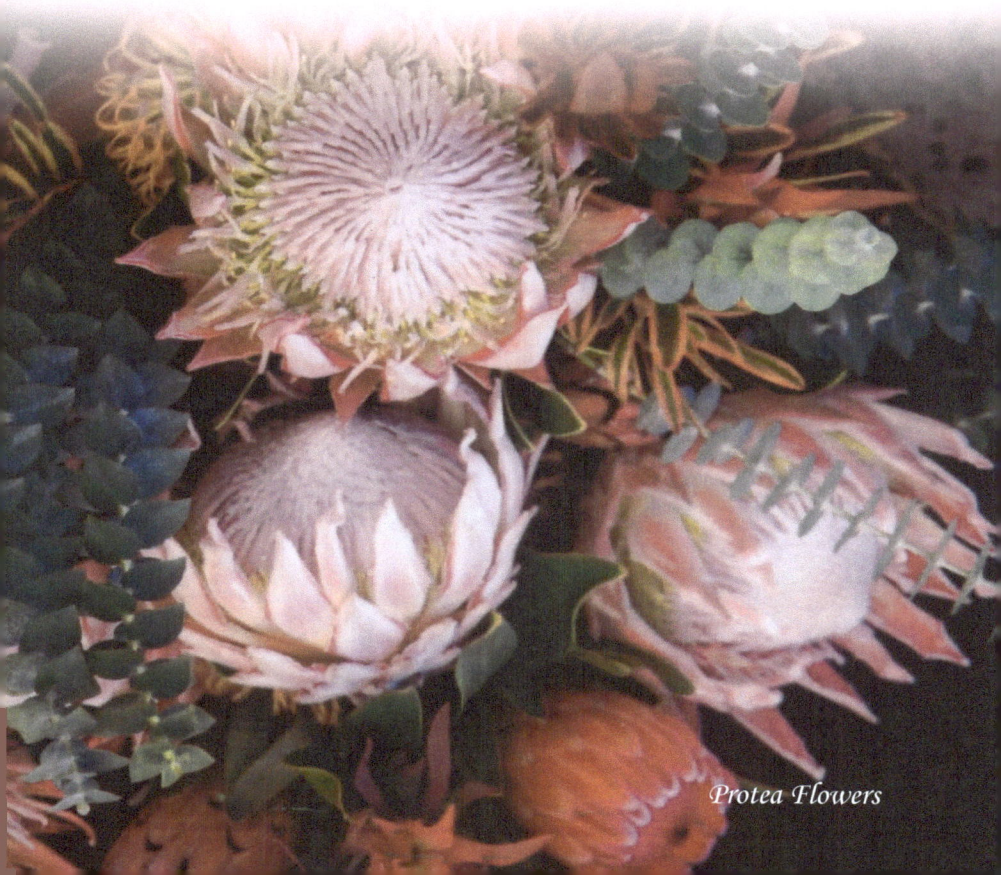

Protea Flowers

Next week, they said when they come for them.
Next week, they said when they come to take them from me
"Next week!"
I said, "I NEED THEM NOW!"

The griefs of my own lie heavy in my breasts!

La`ie Point, O`ahu

In this moment, right now,
I do not know what to do
I do not know how to respond to
all of the griefs that lay heavy in my breasts!

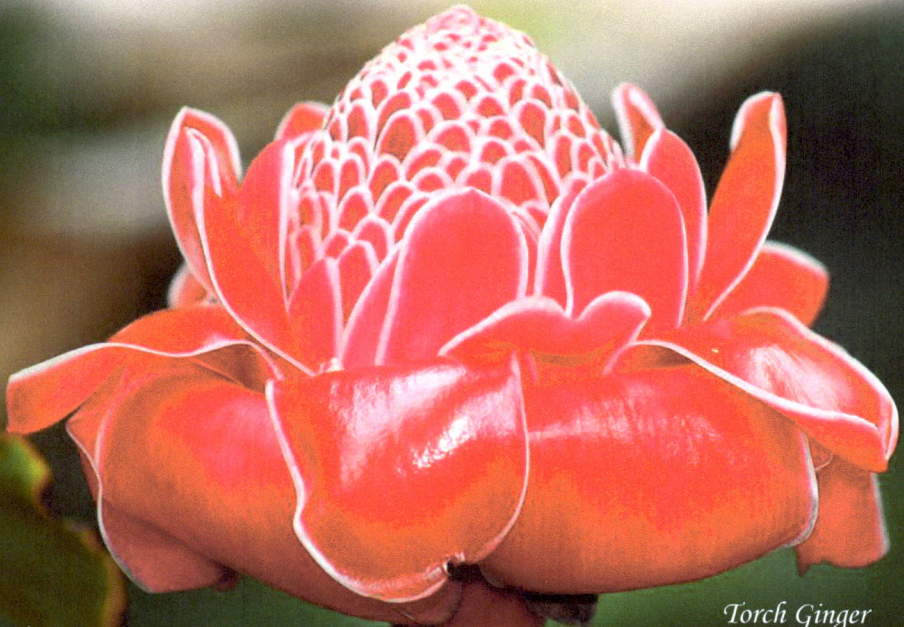

Torch Ginger

You have been my knockers, my doorknobs,
my jugs, my boobs, my bosom, my breasts
since age eight. Men love you, women admire you,
babies suck to quench their thirst, lovers adore you,
kiss and nibble at your delicatessen.

The griefs of my own lie heavy in my breasts!

Ho'omaluhia State Park, O'ahu

Are we star-crossed lovers?
Are we partners in birth and death?
You have been my best friend,
my Sheroes, my confidants.

The griefs of my own lie heavy in my breasts!

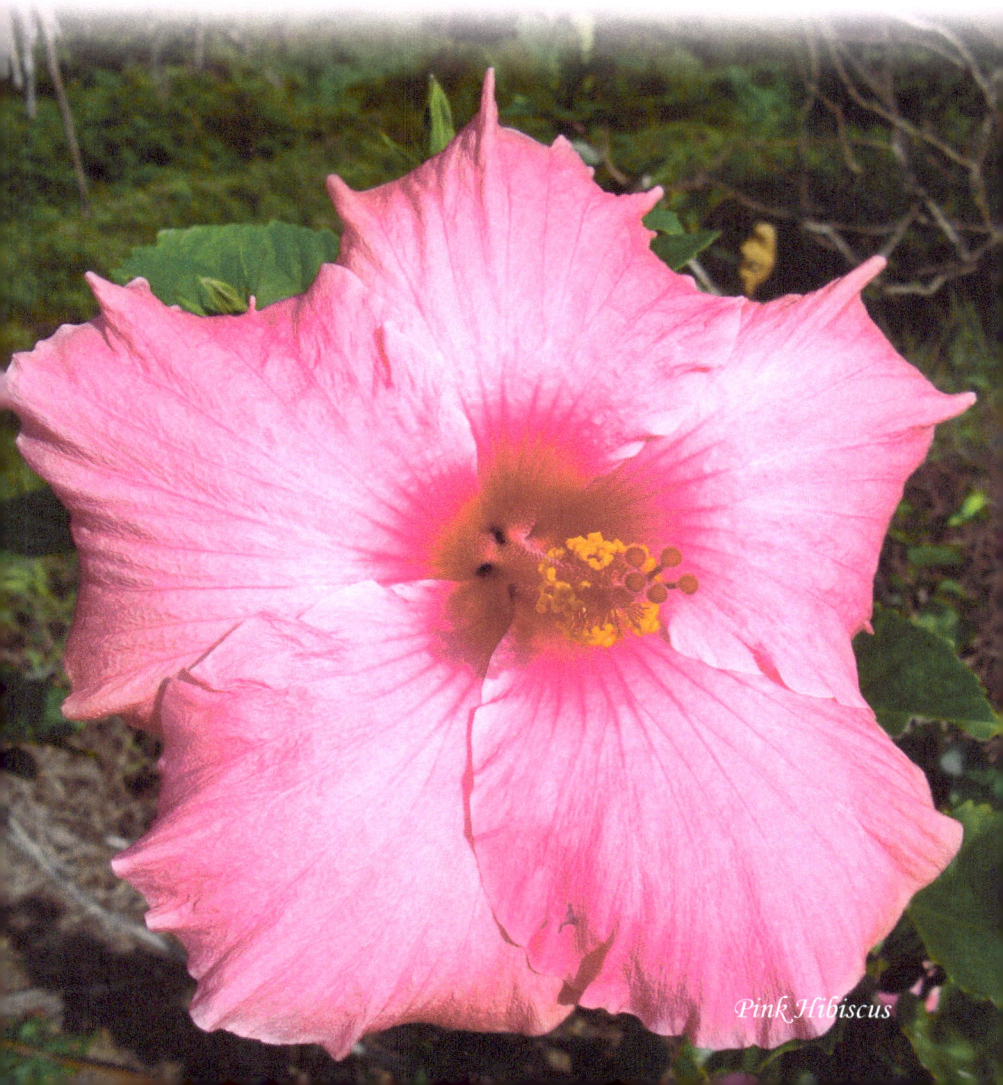

Pink Hibiscus

I wanted to sag with them
I wanted to grow old with them
like a lover who will never leave them faithless,
faithless
even as they fade from fullness.

Sunflowers

I wanted to feel your aging, youth slipping away
sliding quietly into a comfort zone resting on my lap
rocking through our jagged journeys as women:
Black Women, White Women, Asian Women, Hawaiian Women, Pacific
Islander Women, Filipino Women, Muslim Women, Portuguese Women,
Latino Women, Native American Women,
Women of the five continents, victims of the venomous disease.

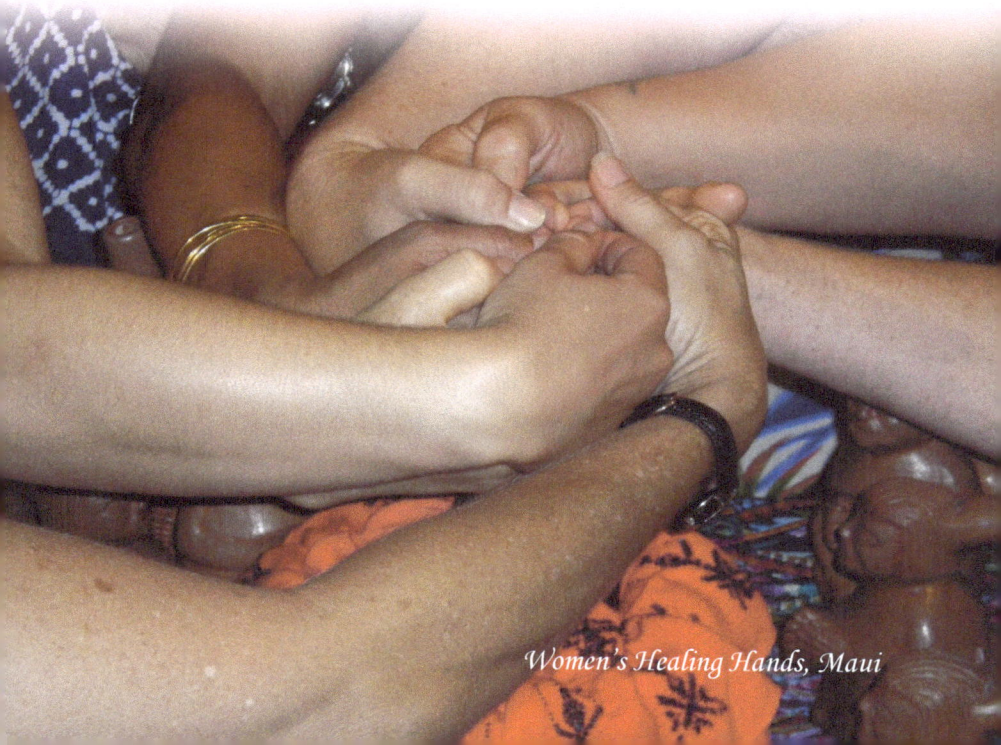

Women's Healing Hands, Maui

Women, crying in the wilderness, adjusting, adjudicating,
promising, processing, progressing, creating,
recreating, releasing, forgiving, accepting, rejecting,
understanding our voices, our powers, as women,
as wives, mothers, sisters, friends, lovers,
sacred
Daughters of the Diaspora.
Nurturing daughters of the Yam.
Daughters of the Womb!

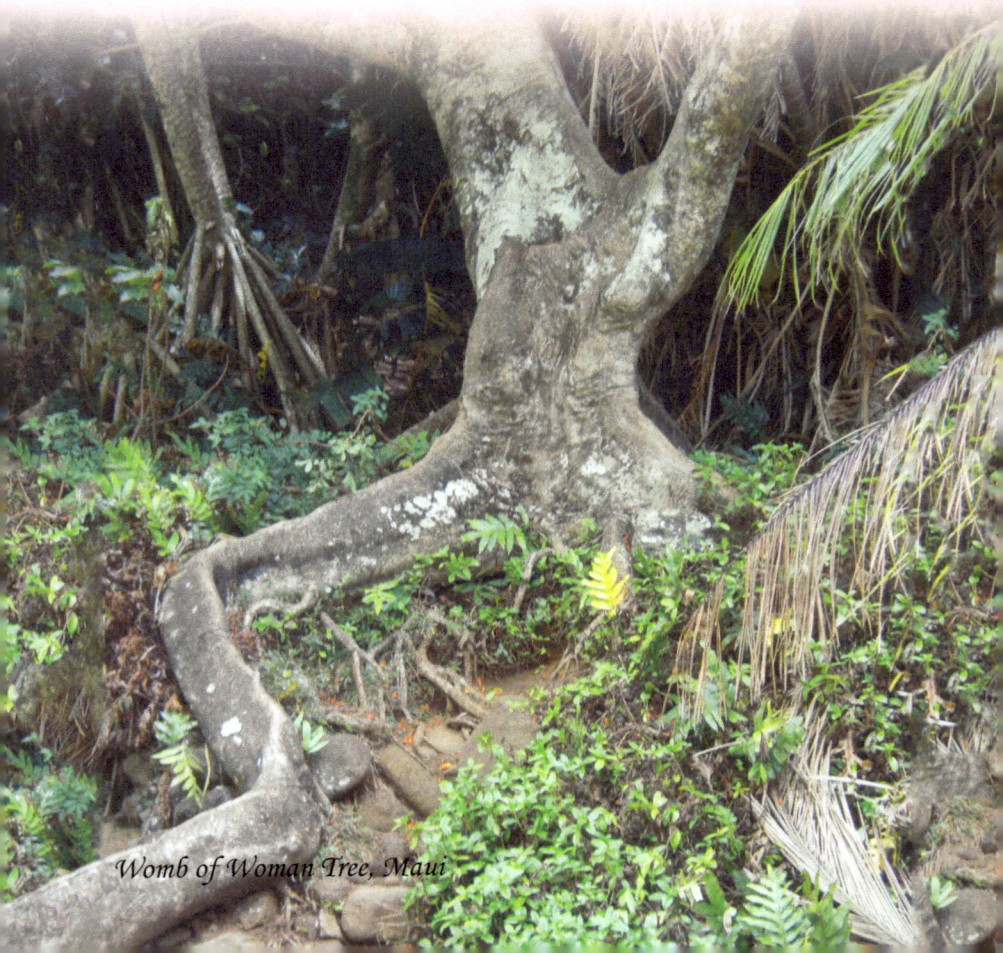

Womb of Woman Tree, Maui

For Ladies only! Pink!
We women wait, in solitude, in patience
In love with our ancestors' spirits!

Our hope!
Our hope for a cure
Our hope for restoration
Our hope for healing
Our hope for the griefs that lie heavy in our hearts!

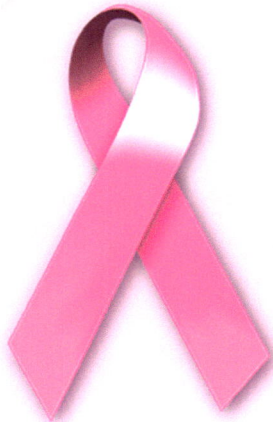

Notes

References

Comprehensive Cancer Information:

National Cancer Institute
www.cancer.gov

American Cancer Society
www.cancer.org

National Cancer Alliance
www.cancersociety.com

American Cancer Society Cancer Action Network
www.ascan.org

Susan G. Komen for the Cure
ww5.komen.org

Hawai`i Affiliate of Susan G. Komen for the Cure
www.komenhawaii.org

www.ingramcontent.com/pod-product-compliance
Lightning Source LLC
Chambersburg PA
CBHW041303290326
41931CB00032B/35